POLICOSANOL

Nature's Answer to High Cholesterol and Clogged Arteries

Candace Salima

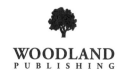

WOODLAND
PUBLISHING

For order information or other inquiries, please contact us:
Woodland Publishing
448 East 800 North
Orem, Utah
84097
Visit us at our web site: www.woodlandpublishing.com
or call us toll-free: (800) 777-2665

The information in this book is for educational purposes only and is not recommended as a means of diagnosing or treating an illness. All matters concerning physical and mental health should be supervised by a health practitioner knowledgeable in treating that particular condition. Neither the publisher nor the author directly or indirectly dispenses medical advice, nor do they prescribe any remedies or assume any responsibility for those who choose to treat themselves.

ISBN 1-58054-395-2
Printed in the United States of America

Contents

Author's Note

My publisher called and asked if I'd be interested in writing a booklet on something called "policosanol." I have to admit, much to my chagrin, I had no idea what it was. Then I started the research. Wow! The man is on to something here.

Nature does indeed have an answer to high cholesterol and its subsequent health issues. As I cruised through the myriad of studies, articles and recommendations from doctors and scientists worldwide I became a believer.

I've broken the booklet down according to the health issues, the policosanol, diet, and last not but least, exercise. I am a big believer that you can take all the supplements in the world and if you refuse to accompany them with a sensible diet and exercise they do you little or no good.

So join me on yet another journey into nature's answer to the pesky health problems that plague mankind.

Let's face facts. Health issues have become a part of everyday life for the bulk of Americans. We simply cannot get away from it. Our diet, our lifestyle, our environment, our genetic code . . . all of these things work against us. There is a proliferation of health issues that plague us, some of which we are going to discuss in length. Why? Because nature has provided us with a little miracle called policosanol. Oh, yeah, even I am completely amazed at the range of health issues policosanol alleviates or prevents. It even has dozens of medical studies to back up the claims.

So, first things first. Let's discuss some health issues that plague almost everyone as they grow older. High cholesterol, heart disease, atherosclerosis, etc. It goes on and on. So, one at a time, here we go.

High Cholesterol

High cholesterol is a condition that strikes a large percentage of Americans today. Cholesterol is a soft, fatty, waxy substance found in the bloodstream and in all the body's cells. A healthy amount of cholesterol is needed for producing cell membranes, some hormones, as well as serving other bodily functions. On the other hand, high levels of cholesterol, known as hypercholesterolemia, creates a major risk for coronary heart disease, which leads to an eventual heart attack.

Cholesterol is produced in two ways. First, your liver produces about 80 percent of the cholesterol in your body, providing the necessary levels for proper bodily functions. Second, you get the rest of the cholesterol, which exists in your system, through the foods you eat. Foods such as meats, poultry, fish, eggs, butter, cheese and whole milk can increase the cholesterol levels in your system. Foods such as fruits, vegetables and cereals, not only have no cholesterol, they help the body metabolize it.

Cholesterol is carried through the blood stream by certain proteins called apolipoproteins. When these proteins wrap around cholesterol and other fats to transport them through your blood system, they then become known as lipoproteins. Lipoproteins are "any member of a group of substances containing both lipid (fat) and protein. They occur in both soluble complexes—as in egg yolk and mammalian blood plasma—and insoluble ones, as in cell membranes. The lipoproteins in blood plasma have been intensively studied because they are the mode of transport for cholesterol (q.v.) through the bloodstream and lymphatic fluid" *(Encyclopedia Britannica)*.

There are four types of these lipoproteins. In their proper balance, they are critical to proper function of the body. Out of balance, they wreak havoc throughout the entire system.

HDL. High-density lipoproteins are very good for your body. High levels of HDL seem to protect against heart attack. Medical experts lean toward the theory that HDL carries cholesterol away from the arteries and back to the liver, where it is passed from the body. Some experts also believe that HDL removes excess cholesterol plaque in the arteries, thus slowing the buildup and preventing heart disease.

In the average man, HDL cholesterol levels range from 40 to 50 mg/dl. In the average woman, they range from 50 to 60 mg/dl. Low HDL cholesterol puts you at a high risk for heart disease. Smoking, obesity and being sedentary can all result in lower HDL cholesterol. If you have low HDL cholesterol, you can help raise it by

- eating whole grains and seeds, such as flax seeds.
- avoiding trans fats and processed foods. (See *Dr. Kenneth Cooper's book Controlling Cholesterol the Natural Way: Eat Your Way to Better Health with New Breakthrough Food Discoveries.*)
- not smoking.
- losing weight or maintaining a healthy weight.
- being physically active for at least thirty to sixty minutes a day on most or all the days of the week.

Progesterone, anabolic steroids and male sex hormones (testosterone) lower HDL cholesterol levels, while female sex hormones (estrogen) raise HDL cholesterol levels.

LDL. Low-density Lipoproteins, on the other hand, can be a ticking time bomb. When too much LDL circulates in the blood, it can slowly build up on the inner walls of the arteries that lead to the heart and brain. Together, with other substances, it can form plaque, a thick, hard deposit that clogs the arteries. This condition is known as atherosclerosis. If a blood clot forms on this plaque it can lead to heart attack or stroke. LDL cholesterol levels of 100 mg/dl is the optimal level of LDL in your bloodstream. With a high level of LDL, more than 160 mg/dl or above, you have two of the high risk factors for cardiovascular disease.

LDL Cholesterol Level Classification

Cholesterol Levels	Level of Health
Less than 100 mg/dl	Optimal
100 to 129 mg/dl	Near Optimal/ Above Optimal
130 to 159 mg/dl	Borderline High
160 to 189 mg/dl	High
190 mg/dl or Higher	Very High

VLDL. Very Low-density Lipoprotein is the most dangerous form of lipoprotein. It carries the least amount of protein and the most amount of fat. VLDL sticks to artery walls and contributes to plaque build-up.

Chylomicrons. Chylomicrons carry only a small percentage of cholesterol through the bloodstream and are rich in another kind of fat called triglycerides.

Triglycerides. Triglycerides are common types of fat (lipids) that are essential to good health when present in normal amounts, less than 150 mg/dl. Abnormally high triglycerides are associated with a number of health conditions such as: cirrhosis (disease of the liver), underactive thyroid (hypothyroidism), poorly controlled diabetes, pancreatitis (inflammation of the pancreas), heart disease, and atherosclerosis.

Proper triglyceride levels, which are critical to maintain, are as follows:

Triglyceride Level Classification

Triglycerides Levels	Level of Risk
Less than 150 mg/dl	Normal
150 to 199 mg/dl	Borderline
200 to 499 mg/dl	High Risk
500 mg/dl or Higher	Very High Risk

Healthy levels of cholesterol as a whole are as follows:

Whole Cholesterol Level Classification

Cholesterol Levels	Level of Risk
Less than 200 mg/dl	Normal
200-239 mg/dl	Borderline High Risk
240 mg/dl or Higher	High Risk

There is good news. Policosanol, further discussed later in this booklet, has been shown in numerous studies to reduce cholesterol. And now, in a recent study, it has been stated that MRIs (Magnetic Resonance Imaging) can accurately track the progress of statin drugs in the treatment of high cholesterol. If it can track the progress of statin drugs, which have a high incidence of negative side effects, it can also track the progress of alternative types of treatment as well. So, should you choose to go the natural route, which should be done under the care of a qualified health professional, you can track your progress very carefully.

Atherosclerosis

Atherosclerosis is the result of fatty substances, cholesterol, cellular waste products, calcium and fibrin (a clotting material in the blood) building up on the inner lining of an artery. The buildup that results is called plaque. In essence, it is the thickening and hardening of arteries. It affects large and medium-sized arteries, although the type of artery where plaque can develop varies with each person.

The American Heart Association says that atherosclerosis or clogged arteries accounts for nearly three-fourths of all deaths from cardiovascular disease.

According to the same study discussed in the cholesterol section: "Our study increases the likelihood that MRI could eventually be used as a predictive technology for determining which patients should be placed on statin therapy for atherosclerosis," said cardiologist Dr. Joao Lima, who led the study.

The following are possible causes of permanent damage to the arteries:

- Elevated levels of cholesterol and triglyceride in the blood.
- High blood pressure and the resulting scarring on inner vessel walls.
- Cigarette smoke.

You guessed it, policosanol helps in this area as well. Keep reading.

Heart Disease

Heart Disease is no picnic. Extensive clinical and statistical studies have identified several factors that increase your risk for heart disease. Some can be changed, some cannot. The more risk factors you have, the greater the risk of heart disease.

There are three major factors that cannot be changed:

Increasing age. Approximately 84 percent of people who die of coronary disease are age sixty-five or older. At older ages, women who have heart attacks are twice as likely as men to die from them within a few weeks.

Male gender. Men have a greater risk of heart attack than women, and they have them earlier in life. Even post-menopausal women, who have an increased death rate from heart disease, are less at risk than men.

Heredity. A family history of coronary heart disease in parents, siblings or offspring is a major risk factor.

And accordingly, there are six factors that can be modified or treated:

Tobacco smoke. Stop smoking! Not only can it give you cancer, if you are a smoker your risk of developing coronary heart disease is two to four times greater than nonsmokers. In addition, smokers are more than ten times likely as nonsmokers to develop peripheral vascular disease.

High blood cholesterol levels. The risk of coronary heart disease and stroke rises as blood cholesterol levels rise. When other factors exist, such as high blood pressure and tobacco use, this increases the risk even more.

High blood pressure. High blood pressure increases the heart's workload, causing it to enlarge and weaken over time. It also increases the risk of congestive heart failure, heart attack, kidney failure, and stroke.

Physical inactivity. Lack of physical activity is another risk factor for coronary heart disease. Exercise can help control blood cholesterol, diabetes, obesity and can lower high blood pressure in some people.

Obesity and overweight. People who have excess body fat are more likely to develop heart disease and stroke, even if they have no other risk factors. Obesity places excess strain on the heart and is directly linked with coronary heart disease because it influences blood pressure, blood cholesterol, triglyceride levels and increases the likelihood of developing diabetes.

Diabetes mellitus. Diabetes severely increases the risk of cardiovascular disease. Three-fourths of people with diabetes die of some form of heart or blood vessel disease.

Additionally, there have been indications that individual response to stress may also be a contributing factor to heart disease.

Luckily, there are several things you can do to counteract the risk factors for heart disease. Following is the American Heart Association's checklist for reducing heart disease risk:

- Have your blood cholesterol checked regularly. If it is high, take appropriate steps to lower it. Suggestions are covered in the following documentation.
- Don't smoke!
- Have your blood pressure checked regularly. Take the appropriate steps to lower it. If it is high, use first natural methods, such as cayenne or mangosteen juice, then moving to prescription drugs as a last resort.
- Be physically active. Take at least thirty minutes of physical activity a minimum of five days a week.

- Recognize and treat diabetes.
- Maintain a healthy weight.
- Eat healthy foods low in saturated fat, cholesterol and sodium. Avoid trans fats at all costs.
- Don't drink too much alcohol; it can increase your blood pressure, not to mention the other multiple health issues that arise from excess drinking of alcoholic beverages.

Some of the main heart diseases are as follows:

Angina is defined as chest pain generally caused by the lack of oxygen from restricted blood flow to the heart. Pain can also be generated to the neck, jaw or arm. Angina is the primary symptom of coronary disease.

Heart attack is defined as scarring, or death, of heart muscle due to lack of oxygen. Oxygen rich blood is blocked by a blood clot in a coronary artery, usually due to the narrowing of the artery, caused by the aggregation of plaque.

Peripheral artery disease (PAD) is the buildup of fatty deposits on the inner lining of the artery walls. These blockages restrict blood circulation mainly to the arteries leading to the kidneys, stomach, arms, legs and feet.

Peripheral vascular disease is the narrowing of blood vessels that carry blood to the arms, legs and kidneys. There are two types of circulation disorders:

- Functional peripheral vascular diseases don't have an organic cause. They don't involve defects in blood vessels' structure. They're usually short-term effects related to "spasm" that may come and go. Reynaud's disease is an example. It can be triggered by cold temperatures, emotional stress, working with vibrating machinery or smoking.
- Organic peripheral vascular diseases are caused by structural changes in the blood vessels, such as inflammation and tissue damage. Peripheral artery disease is an example. It's caused by fatty buildups in arteries that block normal blood flow.

Herpes Simplex Virus

There are three main types of herpes virus. Two of them are type 1 and type 2. Type 1, (herpes simplex) causes cold sores, skin eruptions, and inflammation of the eye cornea. An infected eye can lead to serious complications. Treat it immediately. Type 2 (genital herpes) is the most common form and is a sexually transmitted disease. This virus can be passed onto babies in the birth canal; therefore, a Cesarean section may be required. The virus never leaves the body; it can only be kept under control. If not controlled, it will cause painful blisters around the mouth and genitals, which are highly infectious. Low immunity and stress can cause the dormant virus to break out into open sores.

Fortunately there are two supplements that make a huge difference in the fight against herpes. First, the docosanol alcohol located within policosanol has had some success managing the symptoms. Second, L-lysine, an amino acid, has a huge effect on the herpes simplex virus. These will be discussed at length later on in the booklet.

Platelet Aggregation

Platelets (thrombocytes) are manufactured in the bone marrow. They are the smallest type of blood cells and play a major role in blood coagulation, clotting and hemostasis (stoppage of bleeding). Under normal conditions, platelets will not attach to each other or to the walls of blood vessels. However, an injury will result in the release of activators into the liquid part of blood (plasma), and these activators make the platelets clump together (aggregate) and expand.

Platelets will not attach to the healthy top layer of the interior of the blood vessel. However, they will stick to the second layer if it has been exposed due to injury. As the platelets continue to stick to each other and to the sides of the injured tissue, they form a plug (a blood clot) that becomes covered with strands of thread-like fibrin. Soon the plug shrinks into place and obstructs any further loss of blood. Platelets also release chemicals that begin the healing process.

Prostate Disease

As men age, the prostate may become a source of problems. The three most common problems are inflammation (prostatitis), prostate enlargement (benign prostatic hyperplasia), and prostate cancer. Prostate cancer is the most common type of cancer (excluding skin cancer) among American men. According to the American Cancer Society, men aged fifty and older, and those over the age of forty-five who are in high-risk groups, such as African-American men and men with a family history of prostate cancer, should have a prostate-specific antigen (PSA) blood test and digital rectal exam (DRE) once every year.

The prostate is a small hormone-dependent organ positioned under the urinary bladder that is influenced by the androgen hormones, testosterone and dihydrotestosterone. Under the influence of these hormones, by puberty, the prostate matures and reaches full size and weight by the age of twenty-five. While testosterone has received much attention for contribution towards one's masculinity, its conversion to dihydrotestosterone by the enzyme steroid 5 a-reductase is associated with benign growth of the prostate. Tissues where steroid 5 a-reductase enzyme activity is high such as, the prostate, dihydrotestosterone is believed to be the major active androgen. It is, therefore, critical to address the suppression of steroid 5 a-reductase enzyme in efforts to resolve an enlarged prostate. Adjunct therapy must also focus on nutritional support for the gland, which includes nutrients that enhance blood flow, reduce swelling, balance hormonal disturbances, act as anti-carcinogenic agents and provide for the health of prostate tissue.

Nature's Answer

So what is the answer? The previously mentioned health risks are frightening, there's no question of that. But nature has provided the solution to multiple health issues for millennia. In particular, policosanol has proven to be the golden fleece.

What Is Policosanol?

Before we can get into the who, what, where, why and how of policosanol, we're going to have to delve into the scientific end a little. I know, it can make your head spin, but follow closely, and let's see if we can traverse this rocky path together.

Policosanol is a mixture of long-chain fatty alcohols isolated and refined from plants like sugar cane, rice or a substance such as beeswax. The bulk of medical studies have been conducted on sugar cane policosanols. Although rice and beeswax hold policosanol, there is no guarantee product derived from these other sources will have the same results.

The main ingredient in policosanol is octacosanol, but as "poli" implies, it is actually a mixture of many alcohols including: dotriacontanol, hexacosanol, hexatriacontanol, triacontanol, tetracosanol, tetratriacontanol, and docosanol. It appears to have the potency of statin drugs, which are common medications for those with high cholesterol or heart disease, such as atherosclerosis and coronary artery disease.

As mentioned above, policosanol can come from multiple sources, but the main ones we will discuss will be beeswax policosanol, rice wax policosanol and sugar cane wax policosanol.

Beeswax. There are numerous studies in progress in regards to policosanol from beeswax. Until those studies are complete there is no way to know if this type of policosanol is equal to that from sugar cane. Exercise caution in choosing your policosanol supplement until more is known.

Rice bran wax. The original Japanese research into policosanol was done on the rice wax policosanol. Rice is apparently the richest source of docosanol.

Sugar cane wax. The bulk of medical studies have been conducted in Havana, Cuba, and therefore, have been done on sugar cane wax.

How Can It Benefit You?

Numerous studies have shown policosanol improves cholesterol metabolism and reduces circulating triglycerides. Let's break down the main alcohols in policosanol that have been the subject of multiple studies and see what each one does.

- Docosanol (doe-KOE-san-ole) protects the prostate gland and is considered a primary active component of the herb pygeum africanum, which is used to maintain prostate health. It also comes from the family of antivirals, meaning medical studies have shown some success in the fighting of viruses with docosanol.
- Hexacosanol has been shown to aid in nerve regeneration, as well as inhibit glucose-stimulated insulin secretion.
- Octacosanol has been studied for its effects on improving physical performance and reducing fatigue.
- Triacontanol is a naturally occurring plant hormone that acts as a growth stimulator aiding in cell photosynthesis.

Policosanol has been proven in studies to benefit people in the following ways:

- Inhibits the oxidation of dangerous LDL cholesterol.
- Lowers the damaging LDL cholesterol.
- Increases protective HDL cholesterol levels.
- Does not interfere with sex life, as statin drugs often do.
- Reduces platelet aggregation.
- Improves intermittent claudication (pain in the leg muscles due to inadequate blood supply).
- May prevent and reverse atherosclerotic lesions and thrombosis, although the studies are inconclusive on this matter.
- Does not cure the herpes virus, but it alleviates the symptoms and relieves the pain and suffering. Docosanol, one of the policosanol alcohols, is the only FDA approved compound for the treatment of herpes simplex virus.
- Protects and maintains prostate health.

Another note of interest is the reaction of policosanol on post-menopausal women. The female hormones estrogen and progesterone appear to provide a protective effect against cardiovascular disease. As women go through menopause and hormone levels begin to drop, there is often an elevation of cholesterol and increased risk of cardiovascular disease. The efficacy of policosanol was studied on a group of 224 postmenopausal women with elevated cholesterol. After the eighteen-week course of the randomized, double blind, placebo-controlled study, doctors noted that the group receiving policosanol experienced a 17 percent reduction in total cholesterol, a 25 percent reduction in LDL cholesterol, and a significant rise in HDL cholesterol.

Okay, I don't know about you, but my brain is about burst with the science, so let me share a little about my ancestors. Passed down through multiple generations was a gum salve that was as close to miraculous for healing unlike anything I've ever seen. One of the ingredients, a substantial part of the salve, is beeswax. Suddenly, I'm beginning to realize that the policosanol in the beeswax probably had a great deal to do with the healing process.

How Does It Work?

Although scientists have not quite pinpointed how policosanol works, it has become clear, through multiple studies, that it appears to work by blocking the body's synthesis of cholesterol. In addition to lowering cholesterol, more specifically lowering LDLs, raising HDLs and lowering triglycerides, it aids in preventing heart disease and atherosclerosis.

Policosanol does not inhibit the HMG-CoA enzyme as does the statin drugs normally prescribed for lowering cholesterol. According to the study "Effect of policosanol on lipofundin-induced atherosclerotic lesion in rats" conducted and authored by M. Noa in 1995, there is the possibility that it inhibits a different enzyme. Whatever its mechanism, and whatever the exact chemical interaction, the end result is very exciting. Policosanol has been shown to do naturally what statin drugs do chemically, without the host of side effects like sleep problems, dizziness, muscle aches, muscle weakness, muscle damage (in more severe cases) and reduced sexual function.

Precautions

Policosanol is exceptionally safe. Clinical trails show that elderly persons, diabetics and those with liver damage can safely take policosanol. Although policosanol produced no teratongenic effects in animals, it is not recommended that pregnant and lactating women take policosanol.

Side Effects

The safety of policosanol has been shown in numerous studies conducted on humans and animals. The most frequently reported side effects are weight loss (1.8 percent) of patients treated, polyuria (frequent or excessive urination occurred in 0.7 percent of patients), and headaches (0.6 percent).

In other words, multiple studies have medically proven policosanol to be one of the safest supplements on the market.

Drug Interactions

In short and long-term studies, policosanol has been simultaneously employed with calcium antagonists, beta-blockers and diuretics without evidence of clinically relevant adverse reactions. NASAIDs, anti-depressants, digoxin, warfarin, thyroid hormones, and anti-ulcer drugs have also shown no evidence of clinically relevant adverse interactions.

Dosage Information

Most clinicians familiar with policosanol recommend a beginning dose of 10 mg once a day taken with the evening meal. This is because cholesterol production is higher during sleep. This dosage can increase to 20 mg per day, but higher doses are not recommended until current studies are completed. At these doses, policosanol lowers total cholesterol by 17 percent to 21 percent and LDL by 21 percent to 29 percent, raising HDL by 8 percent to 15 percent. Very promising numbers.

Supplemental Vitamins, Herbs and Enzymes

There are a few things in the world that work better alone, but not very many. If you wish to maintain optimum heart and artery health you can add a couple more supplements to the mix.

Get on a solid multi-vitamin, one which has proven maximum absorption. There are those that absorb in the upper gastrointestinal tract in the first twenty minutes and achieve 90 percent absorption. That is very good. There are others that are powdered and put into a drink and have an excellent absorption rate. Verify the minimum RDAs (Recommended Daily Allowances) have been met or exceeded. If they are exceeded, make sure they have been exceeded safely and for good reason. Do the research, find the vitamin that works best for you for your health, age and sex.

According to a report by the *Journal of the American College of Nutrition,* "We examined 182 participants for selected plasma vitamin concentrations and clinically relevant variables including homocysteine, lipids and LDL-C oxidation indices at baseline and six months . . . We conclude that a multi-ingredient vitamin formula with antioxidant properties has measurable effects on homocysteine and LDL-C oxidation indices."

What does that mean? Well, let me break it down for you. A six month study was conducted to prove or disprove the effectiveness of a highly efficient multi-vitamin in fighting homocysteine, lipids and LDL-C levels. Let me define the words:

- Homocysteine is an amino acid (a building block of protein) produced in the human body. Homocysteine may irritate blood vessels, leading to blockages in the arteries (atherosclerosis).

- Lipids "are any of various substances that are soluble in nonpolar organic solvents (as chloroform and ether), that with proteins and carbohydrates constitute the principal structural components of living cells, and that include fats, waxes, phosphatides, cerebrosides, and related and derived compounds," according to the *Merriam Webster Dictionary*. Triglycerides are lipids, and we've already discussed how abnormally high triglycerides are associated with a number of health conditions such as cirrhosis (disease of the liver), underactive thyroid (hypothyroidism), poorly controlled diabetes, pancreatitis (inflammation of the pancreas), heart disease, and atherosclerosis.

We already know LDLs are bad, bad, bad when they are at high levels in your body. LDL-C simply stands for LDL-cholesterol.

Again, it is important to find and begin faithfully taking a high quality multi-vitamin that has the characteristics of high absorption, good quality control, and the correct levels of nutrients. I'll repeat it one more time, do the research and then act on it. You'll be doing yourself a huge favor.

Individual supplements can be very beneficial although I don't recommend you buy them all and start taking a cocktail. Do a little research, see which ones fit your needs the best and proceed from there.

Alfalfa (Medicago sativa). This herb is beneficial in many ways. The whole herb is used medicinally to help stop bleeding, to benefit the kidneys and as a general tonic. It is a good laxative and a natural diuretic. It is a folk remedy for arthritis and is reputed to be an excellent appetite stimulant. Alfalfa possesses extremely high nutritional value. An excellent source of vitamins A and D, alfalfa leaf is used in the infants' cereal pablum. Also rich in vitamin K, alfalfa leaf has been used in medicine to encourage blood clotting. Alfalfa also lowers blood cholesterol.

Adonis (Adonis vernalis). The leaves and tops of this herb contain a number of biologically active compounds, including cardioactive glycosides that benefit the heart. It dilates the coronary vessels. They are similar to those found in foxglove but gentler. These substances increase the heart's efficiency by increasing its output while slowing its rate. It is also used for mitral stenosis and edema due to heart failure.

Arnica (Arnica montana). Arnica has been used for heart problems (as it contains a cardio-tonic substance), to improve circulation, to reduce cholesterol and to stimulate the central nervous system. But the internal use should only be done under supervision. It displays astonishing stimulating, decongesting and relaxing properties. The heart is both stimulated in deficient conditions and relieved in excess ones, depending on the case presented.

Bilberry (Myrtilli fructus). Studies show bilberry has an effect on heart contractions and blood vessels that is thought to be caused by the berries stimulating the production of prostaglandins. There is evidence that they also help prevent blood clots. Bilberry's high anthocyanin content makes it a potentially valuable treatment for varicose veins, hemorrhoids, and capillary fragility. Bilberries are incorporated into European pharmaceuticals that are used to improve circulation and eye health. Several scientific studies support this use.

Broom (Sarothamnus scoparius, Cytisus scoparius). The ingredient sparteine reduces the heart rate and the isoflavones are estrogenic. Broom is used mainly as a remedy for an irregular, fast heartbeat and to treat cardiac edema. The plant acts on the electrical conductivity of the heart, slowing and regulating the transmission of the impulses.

Coenzyme Q10. Made naturally in the body, coenzyme Q10 is used by cells to produce energy for necessary cell growth and maintenance. In addition, it is a powerful antioxidant that mops up free radicals and prevents damage to the mitochondria. It has also been used, with some success, in battling Parkinson's, specifically in controlling the tremors associated with the disease. Most importantly, coenzyme Q10, coupled with policosanol, seems to benefit the heart greatly. In some studies, using the supplement appeared to lessen chest pain (angina), lower blood pressure and improve the symptoms of heart failure. In and of itself, it also improves the health of the mouth and gums.

Hawthorn berry (Crataegi fructus). Hawthorn has been the subject of a twenty-five year study conducted by a German hospital/medical school. The results were astounding. Historically, the hawthorn berry was used as a cardiac tonic, for edema, heart attack, to regulate blood pressure, for arteriosclerosis, inflamed heart muscle, for rapid or arrhythmic heartbeat, for a weak pulse, dropsy and heart murmurs. In Germany, they discovered it to be one of the most powerful nutrients for the heart on the earth. Add this to the policosanol supplement you are taking and you cannot go wrong.

Hawthorn berry and coenzyme Q10 have shown no propensity for interfering with medications currently being taken by heart and cholesterol patients. However, consult with your doctor to insure there is no known interference.

Lily of the Valley (Convallaria majalis). Lily of the valley is perhaps the most valuable heart remedy used today. It is used for nervous sensitivity, neurasthenia, apoplexy, epilepsy, dropsy, valvular heart diseases, heart pains and heart diseases in general. It has an action equivalent to foxglove without its potential toxic effects. Lily of the valley may be used in the treatment of heart failure and water retention where this is associated with the heart. It will aid the body where there is difficulty with breathing due to congestive conditions of the heart. Also used for arteriosclerosis with angina and arterial hypotension. Lily of the valley encourages the heart to beat more slowly, regularly and efficiently. It is also strongly diuretic, reducing blood volume and lowering blood pressure. It is better tolerated than foxglove, since it does not accumulate within the body to the same degree. Relatively low doses are required to support heart rate and rhythm, and to increase urine production.

L-lysine. And essential amino acid, L-lysine is of the branched-chain amino acids. A useful aspect of this amino acid is its ability to fight cold sores and the herpes viruses. When the amount of lysine present within the body exceeds the amount of arginine, the growth of the herpes virus is inhibited. Taking L-lysine together with vitamin C with bioflavonoids, can effectively fight and/or prevent herpes outbreaks.

Do not take lysine for longer than six months at a time.

Mistletoe (Visci albi). The European variety of mistletoe is chiefly used to lower blood pressure and heart rate, ease anxiety and promote sleep. This, in relation to the heart is a wonderful thing. Mistletoe's efficacy as an anti-cancer treatment has been subject to a significant amount of research. Studies going back twenty-five years show mistletoe impairs the growth of test-tube tumor cells. In Germany three mistletoe-based chemotherapy agents are administered by injection to treat human cancers. The great advantage offered by mistletoe extracts is that unlike other chemotherapeutic drugs, their immunostimulant and tonic effects are nontoxic and well tolerated. There is no doubt that certain constituents, especially the viscotoxins, exhibit an anti-cancer activity, but the value of the whole plant in cancer treatment is still not fully accepted.

Mistletoe should *never*, under any circumstances, be taken by a pregnant woman, as it is a contraindicator. In other words, it stimulates the uterus and will cause spontaneous miscarriage.

Motherwort (Leonurus cardiaca). Motherwort is primarily an herb of the heart. Several species have sedative effects, decreasing muscle spasms and temporarily lowering blood pressure. Chinese studies found that extracts decrease clotting and the level of fat in the blood and can slow heart palpitations and rapid heartbeat.

Myrrh (Myrrha). Used to increase circulation and stimulate the flow of blood to the capillaries, myrrh also clears out mucus-clogged passages throughout the body. Antiseptic to mucus membranes, myrrh regulates secretions of these tissues. Research suggests that myrrh can lower blood cholesterol levels. In China, it is taken to move blood and relieve painful swellings.

Pygeum africanum. Belonging to the Rosaceae family, *Pygeum africanum* is an evergreen tree native to the southern regions of Africa: Madagascar, Cameroon, and Central Africa. Much of the clinical and pharmacological studies have focused on bark extracts of africanum for the treatment of benign prostatic hypertropghy (BPH). Specifically, three classes of compounds endowed with biological synergistic activity have demonstrated anti-BPH activity. The phytosterols (beta-sistosterol) possess anti-inflammatory properties that are mediated by inhibition of prostaglandins biosynthesis. The prostaglandin content is considerably increased in patients with BPH. Pentacyclic triterpenes are another class of compounds characterized by anti-edema activity, a common occurrence during inflammation. A third class of compounds, known as ferulic esters, consist of docosanol and tetracosanol. These esters are endowed with anticholesterolemic activity both at the blood and prostate level. It is well known that in BPH there is an accumulation of cholesterol and its metabolites, which can participate in androgen metabolism (i.e. testosterone synthesis). In both animal and human studies, subjects have had significant greater improvement in both BPH and prostatitis with no side effects.

Saw palmetto (Sabal fructus). Shown to prevent the conversion of testosterone to dihydrotestosterone (DHT), saw palmetto extract also inhibits DHT binding to cellular and nuclear receptor sites, thereby increasing the metabolism and excretion of DHT. A double-blind placebo-controlled study evaluated the hormonal effects of saw palmetto extract given to men with benign prostatic hypertrophy (BPH) for three months prior to operation. The study found that saw palmetto displayed an estrogenic and antiprogesterone effect as determined by estrogen and progesterone receptor activity. It successfully treats enlarged and weakened prostate as well as impotence.

Zinc. Found in every cell of the body, zinc, in fact, functions in more enzymatic reactions than any other mineral. Tissues with high concentrations of zinc include the bone, skin, kidney, liver, pancreas, retina, and the prostate. Zinc, as it relates to prostate function, is crucial and a deficiency may be a contributing factor in prostate enlargement. Zinc intake has been shown to reduce the size of the prostate and to reduce symptomology in the majority of patients.

Exercise

Exercise, one of the longest four letter words in the history of mankind. Of course, there are those who live to exercise. They spend hours in the gym, pool, courts and or on the fields of competition . . . then there are the rest of us. Struggling to meet deadlines, keep the boss happy, feed the hubby and kids, keep the housework up to speed, the garden producing, the family happy, church or civic duties completed, it goes on and on. In the midst of all that we are actually supposed to exercise too.

Well, we need to. If we hope to live long, healthy lives, exercise has to come into play, even if it means only a daily walk. Let's start with the basics the American Heart Association has laid out.

- Wear comfortable clothes and sneakers or flat shoes with laces.
- Begin slowly. Gradually build up to thirty to sixty minutes of activity daily. You can divide those into two fifteen-minute sessions, or two thirty-minute sessions.
- Exercise at the same time every day so that it becomes a natural part of your routine.
- Drink 8 ounces of filtered or bottled water before exercising.
- Exercise with a friend or family member, you'll be more likely to stick to it.
- Note your activities in a logbook or journal. Write down the distance or length of time of activity and how you feel after each session. If you miss a day, plan a make-up day or add fifteen minutes to your next session.
- Use variety to keep your interest. Walk one day, swim the next, go for a bike ride or play an active sport like basketball.
- Join an exercise group, health club or the YMCA. Remember to clear your intended exercise program with your health care professional first.
- Look for chances to be more active during the day. Walk the mall before shopping, park further out, take the stairs rather than the escalator or elevator, or take ten to fifteen minute walking breaks while watching TV or sitting for extended periods of time.
- Don't get discouraged if you stop exercising for awhile. Just start again and work your way back up gradually.
- Don't exercise right after meals, when it's hot or very humid, or when you are feeling under the weather.

Exercise Journal

Let's keep it simple. You can use something as simple as a notebook or go fancy and buy an exercise diary from the store. But the main things you need to keep track of are:

- Your activities. For instance, walking, swimming, weightlifting, yoga, etc.
- How often you do each of these activities.

- How long you do these activities.
- Inches/weight lost.
- Overall general health. Are you feeling better? Do you have more energy?

If you will track these diligently, you will find that it will provide the impetus to keep exercising. Just as goals are reach more easily, if they are written down, so to is progress.

Suggested Beneficial Exercises

Stress is a high factor in the average American's life. Because we are constantly on the run, under deadline, not to mention personal pressure, it behooves each of us to find an exercise that releases or eliminates stress. Two programs I have found benefit greatly in that area are yoga and tai chi.

Yoga. Regardless of whether you can appreciate the philosophies behind yoga (I'm not one of those), I cannot deny the physical and psychological benefits of yoga. The simple stretching and breathing exercises eliminate a great deal of stress. This is something that is low impact with maximum benefit. Now, while I cannot stretch myself into a pretzel, I still gain benefit from the simple movements.

Tai chi. Tai chi is a Chinese martial art that is primarily practiced for its health benefits, including a means of dealing with tension and stress.

Tai chi emphasizes complete relaxation, and is essentially a form of meditation, or what has been called "meditation in motion." Unlike the hard martial arts, tai chi is characterized by soft, slow, flowing movements that emphasize force, rather than brute strength. Though it is soft, slow, and flowing, the movements are executed precisely.

Tai chi and yoga have been shown to aid in healing or gaining relief from arthritis, rheumatism, balance improvement, high blood pressure, post-operative recovery, post-traumatic stress, stress reduction, athletic performance, issues of aging, and weight management.

Diet

Food, my favorite thing. Familial memories go way back, most of them centered around Sunday dinner and the sumptuous meals my mother put together. As our society has become more sedentary, we are experiencing a resulting epidemic of obesity. The meals of yesteryear are now centering around our stomachs, bottoms and thighs. It's a fact of life, that our diet must change to fit our lifestyles. You know the lifestyles I'm talking about, office workers, school teachers, students, scientists, doctors, etc. We no longer have to scrape and scramble to put food on the table. The larger part of America no longer farms or ranches, no longer produces gardens, no longer understands that food does indeed come from the heart of the earth. The bulk of our society spends all its time indoors, and we have poor health as a result.

Studies have shown that cholesterol levels are also linked to dietary fats. In particular, trans fats, common in potato chips, french fries and other snack foods and fast foods, are most dangerous to normal cholesterol levels and optimum heart health. Trans fats increase the levels of LDL (bad cholesterol) and lower the levels of HDL (good cholesterol). This should be of particular concern, because trans fats prolong the shelf life of food and are used in far too many foods today. In 2003, the Food & Drug Administration (FDA), announced that all manufacturers will have to list the amount of trans fats in each of their products. For more information on this, check out the FDA's web site at www.fda.gov.

It has always reflected good sense to have a well balanced diet. With the varying trends of high protein/low carbohydrate or high carbohydrate/low protein, all vegetables and fruits/no meats, all meats/no fruits and vegetables, no solid food at all/drink this concoction, and with the myriad of diet supplements there is good cause for worry about America's physical health as a whole.

If you have particular concern for heart health, you can do nothing better than going to the American Heart Association's website for dietary guidelines. Delicious Decisions—the American Heart Association's web site for recipes and dietary tips located at www.deliciousdecisions.org contains a plethora of information and recipes for the heart health conscious individual.

For your average individual, keep your calories at a decent level. Here are simple daily guidelines according to the American Heart Association:

- Watch your caloric intake by eating a wide variety of foods low in saturated fat and cholesterol.
- Eat at least five servings of fruits and vegetables daily.
- Eat poultry and fish without skin, as well as leaner cuts of meat.
- Eat fat-free or 1 percent milk dairy products rather than whole milk dairy products.

Remember, that protein is critical to your diet. You cannot metabolize natural sugars without protein. For instance, if you want to drink two or three glasses of delicious ruby red grapefruit juice, you will have the sugar shakes within the hour. If, however, you eat an egg and a piece of whole wheat toast, there will be no problem with drinking the juice. Use common sense in applying the standards of any organization recommending dietary restrictions.

In other words, be smart. Balance your proteins and carbohydrates without going overboard on either one. I've found *The Zone Diet*, if you must follow one, to be the most sensible with highest degree of benefit and lowest degree of negative results.

Another high quality diet for the cholesterol conscious individual is Dr. Kenneth Cooper's high cholesterol diet. In his book, *Controlling Cholesterol the Natural Way: Eat Your Way to Better Health with New Breakthrough Food Discoveries* details the path to prevention and control of high cholesterol. For more information on Dr. Cooper's established and widely recognized methods of diet, exercise and supplementation, go to www.cooperwellness.com.

Conclusion

The health conscious lifestyle is one that will provide a great many benefits, a longer and healthier life, as well as a better quality of life. It can be very confusing with every Tom, Dick and Harry pouring information onto the information highway, countless books, diets, exercise plans . . . it goes on and on.

The most important thing you can do is to take what you've learned in this booklet and expand on it. There are ways in which you can enjoy health and still have the quality and texture of life you desire. I urge you to not let this booklet be the last you read or study on the topic of policosanol, cholesterol, atherosclerosis, heart disease and so on. It is time to take your health out of the hands of people who don't know you and into your own. Make your doctor your partner, learning all you can about health issues you face. You will find that, armed with knowledge, you are in a much better position to take on all health challenges that come your way.

Good luck . . . I'm on my way to buy some policosanol.

References

Almada, Anthony. "Cuban Lipid Crisis." Nov 2001. *Nutrition Science News.*

American Heart Association: www.americanheart.org

Azzouz M, Kenel PF, Warter J-M, et al. "Enhancement of mouse sciatic nerve regeneration by the long-chain fatty acid, n-hexacosanol." *Exp Neurol.* 1996; 138:189-197.

Balch, James F. M.D. and Balch, Phyllis A. C.N.C. *Prescription for Nutritional Healing*, Second Edition, Avery Publishing Group. 1997 p. 40,317-318.

Castano G, Mas Ferreiro R, Fernandez L, Gamez R, Illnait J, Fernandez C. "A long-term study of policosanol in the treatment of intermittent claudication." Medical Surgical Research Center, Havana City, Cuba. *Aniology* 2001 Feb;52(2):115-25.

Damge C, Hillaire-Buys D, Koenig M, et al. "Effect of n-hexacosanol on insulin secretion in the rat." *Eur J Pharmacol.* 1995; 274:133-139.

Earnest, Conrad P. "Complex Multivitamin Supplementation Improves Homocysteine and Resistance to LDL-C Oxidation." The Cooper Institute. *Journal fo the American College of Nutrition.* vol. 22, No. 5, 400–407 (2003).

Fernandez, J.C., Mas, R. "Comparison of the Efficacy, Safety and

Tolerability of Policosanol versus Fluvastatin in Elderly Hypercholesterolaemic Women." National Center for Scientific Research, Havana City, Cuba. *Clin Drug Invest* 21(2):103-133, 2001.

Harding, Anne. "Buzz on Cholesterol-Lowering Beeswax is Promising." Reuter's Health

Ingels, Darin N.D. "Policosanol Helps Reduce High Cholesterol." 2002-06-06011:00:0, Healthnotes, Inc.

Mas R., Rivas P., Iaquierdo J.E. "A Close Look at Coenzyme Q10 and Policosanol: Pharmacoepidemiologic study of policosanol." *Harvard Heart Letter.* 1999;60:458-67

MRI scan can monitor cholesterol health—study, Reuters, Cardiovascular News Center, Oct 2004, HeartCenterOnline.

Noa, M., Mas, R., de la Rosa, M.C., Magraner J. "Effect of policosanol on lipofundin-induced atherosclerotic lesions in rats." *J Pharm Pharmacol.* 1995 Apr;47(4):289-91.

Yam Cher Seng. "Coenzyme Q10 May Slow the Progression of Parkinsons." Nov 2003. *The New Straits Times*

Woodland Health Series

*Definitive Natural Health Information
At Your Fingertips!*

The Woodland Health Series offers a comprehensive array of single topic booklets, covering subjects from fibromyalgia to green tea to acupressure. If you enjoyed this title, look for other WHS titles at your local health-food store, or contact us. Complete and mail (or fax) us the coupon below and receive the complete Woodland catalog and order form—free!

Or . . .

- Call us toll-free at (800) 777-2665
- Visit our website
  (www.woodlandpublishing.com)
- Fax the coupon (and other correspondence) to
  (801) 334-1913

The Natural Choice for Prostate Health

Saw Palmetto

Immune and Stamina Booster

Cordyceps Sinensis

Rita Gilbert Udall

Potent Soy Isoflavone

Genistein

Rita Elkins, M.H.